The Female Body
BLUEPRINT

A Guide to Understanding
Hormones and Thyroid Health

By: Josh and Jeanne Rubin

www.eastwesthealing.com

Copyright © 2015 Josh and Jeanne Rubin
Published by ✒ Archangel Ink

ISBN: 1942761171
ISBN-13: 978-1-942761-17-4

Table of Contents

Introduction 4

The Estrogen Equation 6

Infertility 15

Menopause 20

Metabolism 25

Food & Nutrition 32

Stress 38

Sleep 47

Exercise 54

Detoxification 57

Conclusion 66

Thank You 68

The Next Step 69

About the Authors 71

Introduction

In 1960, birth control pills were approved for contraceptive use. Since that time, there have been huge changes in our environment and in our lifestyles. Our food is dirty, our water is dirty, and our air is polluted. We work more, spend more, have more debt, don't sleep, never rest, and are always playing catch-up.

Perhaps not surprisingly, in that same time frame, we have seen a dramatic rise in female-related illnesses. In a way, we can say that we are witnessing the results of a 40-year study in which the effects of birth control—along with other environmental factors—are proving detrimental.

To give you some idea of the afflictions affecting women today:

- The average age for puberty has dropped abruptly to 10 years of age.
- Endometriosis, one of the top three causes of female infertility, affects more than 5.5 million women.
- 75% of all women suffer with some premenstrual syndrome symptoms.
- 80% of all women have uterine fibroids. Hysterectomies are performed on 170,000- 300,000 women annually due to uterine fibroids.

- Dysmenorrhea affects approximately 40-70% of women of reproductive age, of which 10% describe severe symptoms.
- Amenorrhea affects 25-60% of female athletes, 25% of runners, and 1.8 to 5% of the population.

Chances are that you have been affected by one or more of the above, especially if you've picked up this book. You've also likely visited a medical professional in hopes of clearing up your female health issues once and for all. But did you walk away with improved health?

Medicine today has been divided into specialties. With the creation of specialties came the inevitable "female" doctors—OB/GYNs. It's easy to think that all afflictions only experienced by women, like the ailments listed above, could be solved by your regular gynecologist or obstetrician, but unfortunately, as is the case with all other medical specialties, most of these doctors aren't looking at the bigger picture. What that means for you is that when you go in to discuss menstrual cramps or PMS, you'll be given birth control pills. If you go in complaining of infertility, you'll be sent to yet another specialist—a fertility specialist—who will pump your body full of hormones. If you complain of depression, you'll likely be sent away with anti-depressants.

There has to be a better way.

Our aim with this book is to start to connect the dots between the major health issues facing women today. We'll look at the relationship between two vital hormones—estrogen and progesterone—and how they interact with the body as a whole. Also vital to this discussion of women's health are the topics of metabolism, nutrition, stress, sleep, exercise, and detoxification, all of which we'll explore in great detail. We'll be looking at your *whole* body to come up with a blueprint that you can follow for the rest of your life to enjoy more energy, fewer symptoms, and vibrant health.

Without further ado, let's get started so you can begin your healing journey today!

The Estrogen Equation

Estrogen and progesterone are the two primary hormones responsible for regulating the female menstrual cycle. Estrogen works during the "building" stage of the menstrual cycle (increasing the uterine lining) and progesterone signals the body to slough off the lining if an egg is not implanted. Estrogen and progesterone constantly work together to maintain optimal balance in our body at all times.

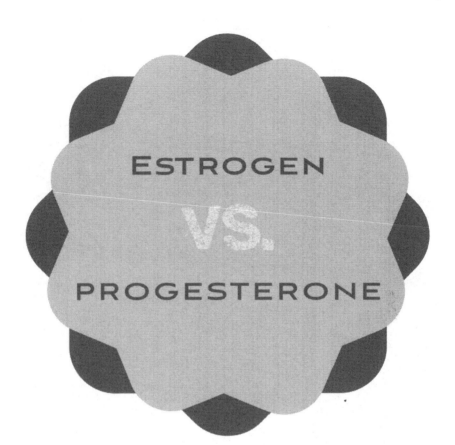

Estrogen

Procreation effects:

- Creates proliferative endometrium
- Necessary for proper ovulation
- Decreases sex drive

Intrinsic effects:

- Causes breast stimulation
- Increases body fat
- Salt and fluid retention
- Depression and headaches
- Interferes with thyroid hormone
- Increases blood clotting
- Impairs blood sugar control
- Loss of zinc and retention of copper
- Reduces oxygen levels in all cells
- Slightly restrains osteoclast (bone loss) function
- Reduces vascular tone
- Increases risk of endometrial cancer
- Increases risk of breast cancer
- Increases risk of gallbladder disease
- Increases risk of autoimmune disorders

Progesterone

Procreation effects:

- Maintains secretory endometrium
- Necessary for survival of embryo
- Restores sex drive

Intrinsic effects:

- Protects against fibrocystic breasts
- Helps use fat for energy
- Natural diuretic
- Natural antidepressant
- Facilitates thyroid hormone action
- Normalizes blood clotting
- Normalizes blood sugar levels
- Normalizes zinc and copper levels
- Restores proper cell oxygen levels
- Stimulates osteoblast bone building
- Restores normal vascular tone
- Prevents endometrial cancer
- Helps prevent breast cancer
- Protects against ovarian cancer
- Restores normal sleep patterns
- Skin moisturizer
- Precursor of corticosteroids

Both hormones are produced in the ovaries, the adrenal glands, and the placenta, and are stored in adipose tissue (fat cells), but we are much more susceptible to estrogen dominance than progesterone dominance. So what is estrogen dominance and why is it a problem for women today?

The term estrogen dominance, as you might guess, is used to describe a state in which the ratio of estrogen to progesterone is skewed too much toward the estrogen side of things. Symptoms of estrogen dominance and progesterone deficiency include:

- Severe cramping
- Heavy bleeding and clotting
- Fibroids
- Endometriosis
- PCOS Polycystic Ovarian Syndrome
- Fibrocystic breasts
- Tender and/or swollen breasts
- Swelling and bloating
- Mood swings
- Memory loss
- Weight gain
- Foggy thinking
- Gallbladder disease
- Hair loss
- Irritability
- Osteoporosis
- Slow metabolism or hypothyroidism
- Insomnia
- Mineral imbalance/deficiency
- Fatigue
- PMS
- Headaches
- Hypoglycemia

Any of that sound familiar? Unfortunately, estrogen dominance is becoming more and more common as our environment and lifestyle continue to evolve in an unbalanced way.

Top Nine Causes of Estrogen Dominance:

1. **Stress of any type.** The body has one response to stress, and it's your nervous system that makes the call on what your body interprets as stress. Exercise (too much or too little), poor eating habits, poor time management, emotional stressors, physical stressors, and environment can all play a role.
2. **Aging.** The ability to produce protective hormones such as progesterone and pregnenolone decreases as we age while estrogen increases.
3. **The inability of the liver to detoxify estrogen when under-nourished.** A protein deficiency, by suppressing liver function, can increase estrogen.
4. **Exogenous sources such as plastics and other xenoestrogens.** Human fertility has declined over the past 20 years as a result of industrial pollutants with estrogen-like effects.
5. **Birth control pills:** Estrogen contraceptives do not prevent conception; they prevent implantation of the embryo into the uterus.[1]
6. **Obesity:** In postmenopausal women, obesity causes the body to increase its production of estrogen through our fats cells, further perpetuating inflammation and other metabolic dysfunctions.
7. **Hysterectomy.** Adrenal and pancreatic problems often arise following the induction of menopause with surgery. Any time there is an organ removed, the remaining organs try frantically to take over some of the removed organ's

---

[1] Dr. John Lee MD "Another problem with the BCP is that it creates a state of anovulation (lack of ovulation), which blocks the ovaries natural production of hormones, including progesterone, with all its protective qualities." Estrogen creates a hypoxic environment, especially at the cellular level. Estrogen causes increased and constant stimulation of the adrenal cortex, which in a chronic state, will decrease sex drive as one is in survival mode.

functions. Additionally, most women are not aware of their choices following a hysterectomy, and certain side effects often lead to hormone therapy.
8. **Premenopause:** Early follicular depletion leading to anovulatory cycles.
9. **Unsaturated fats.** PUFA's (polyunsaturated fatty acids—primarily found in "vegetable" and seed oils), as are found in abundance in the modern diet, are immunosuppressive, anti-thyroid, pro-diabetes, inhibit cellular respiration, and promote the actions of estrogen and cortisol.

Estrogen Production: The Nitty-Gritty

Cholesterol is the basic building block for steroidal hormones. The manufacturing of steroidal hormones from cholesterol takes place in tiny energy packets called mitochondria. Mitochondria are found within every cell of the body except red blood cells.

Thyroid hormone, vitamin A, and other vitamins and minerals are essential in the conversion of cholesterol into pregnenolone. Pregnenolone metabolizes into progesterone and DHEA. DHEA forms DHEA-S (typically measured in labs due to its increased stability), testosterone, and the three estrogens: estrone (E1), estradiol (E2), and estriol (E3). Progesterone is the precursor to both cortisol and the mineral corticoid aldosterone.

In a metabolically healthy and well-nourished body, the formation of pregnenolone from cholesterol is efficient and minimizes the need for cortisol by inhibiting ACTH.

Cortisol is synthesized by progesterone and released by the adrenal glands in response to stress. Although a normal physiological response, chronic stress results in altered hormonal pathways and vitamin and mineral deficiencies.

Deficiencies in thyroid hormone, Vitamin A, light, Vitamin E, and copper decrease the conversion of pregnenolone and progesterone, stimulating the production of cortisol, DHEA, and other androgens. When a system is more heavily compromised and has low resilience to stress, the system is only capable of sustaining cortisol and aldosterone production, leading to degenerative problems, progesterone deficiencies, and estrogen excesses.

In addition to the class of hormones with estrus-like properties, there are also other forms of estrogen found outside the body. These include phytoestrogens, xenoestrogens, and synthetic forms of estrogen. These environmental estrogens are of a growing concern due to their high level of potency and ability to bind to estrogen receptor sites. We'll take a look at these in a later chapter.

Estrogen and Stress

> *"Estrogen offers no physiological benefits other than that of reproduction, and even in reproduction, estrogen's 'shock' effect must be tightly regulated by a well-balanced body."*
>
> – Ray Peat, PhD

We're hearing more and more about the stress hormone cortisol and its effect on health, especially on body weight. Lesser known is the similar effect that excess estrogen can have. Estrogen mimics the shock phase of the stress response and, when left unopposed by progesterone, greatly contributes to:

- Suppression of the thyroid
- Low body temperature and pulse
- Breakdown of fatty acids and protein tissue for energy
- Increased blood pressure
- Inability to store glycogen in the liver
- Blood sugar dysregulation
- Decreased blood volume
- Increased vasoconstriction

It's a vicious cycle—stress can lead to estrogen dominance, and estrogen can lead to more stress on the body. Luckily, the second half of this book is dedicated to teaching you how to reduce estrogen dominance and reclaim balance in your body.

For now, though, let's take a look at two common female health issues and how hormone balance plays a role in each. Just by looking at these two examples—infertility and hot flashes during menopause—we can begin to see the parallels and expand the conclusions to include other female health issues.

Infertility

According to the statistics of the Centers for Disease Control and Prevention (CDC), these are the most recent trends in infertility issues across the country:

- Number of women ages 15-44 with impaired fecundity (impaired ability to have children): 6.7 million
- Percent of women ages 15-44 with impaired fecundity: 10.9%
- Number of married women ages 15-44 that are infertile (unable to get pregnant for at least twelve consecutive months): 1.5 million
- Percent of married women ages 15-44 that are infertile: 6.0%
- Number of women ages 15-44 who have ever used infertility services: 7.4 million

Due to the lack of data in the 1970s (when the first child conceived from IVF was born), whether the infertility epidemic is increasing or decreasing cannot be soundly determined. However, in clinical practice we have seen an astonishing number of couples suffering with infertility issues. Dr. John Lee, international authority and pioneer in the use of natural progesterone cream and natural hormone balance, relayed in one of his presentations that PMS symptoms were not as common "back in the day" and could be easily remedied with proper nutrition and hormone supplementation. He shared that as years went on, PMS symptoms and other female hormone related issues, including infertility, greatly increased.

Mainstream thinking has led many individuals to believe they are unable to get pregnant due to aged ova. Fortunately, there have been many studies proving that the ovaries do not "run out of eggs." In his article "Menopause and its causes," Ray Peat states, "There was never really any basis for that ridiculous belief. Many people just said it, the way they said 'old eggs' (but never old sperm) were responsible for birth defects, or that 'estrogen is the female hormone,' a deficiency of which is the cause of menopausal infertility."

Left and right, people are being led to believe that they are incapable of getting pregnant, so we think it is worth taking the time to explore some other possibilities. What if the inability to conceive is because the uterine environment is not suitable for implantation? And what if this environment was reflective of lifestyle and its influence over physiology?

We encourage this exploration because we have worked with several individuals who have been through a tremendous amount of emotional and financial distress and have found success through nutrition and lifestyle alone!

According to Ray Peat, PhD, "Professor Soderwall and his students at the University of Oregon had shown that the corpora lutea (area of the ovary that mainly produces progesterone) appeared to be failing in aging hamsters, and that Vitamin E supplements could extend fertility by a significant amount. His group showed that the 'aged ova' were not responsible for infertility, but rather that the uterine environment was not suitable for implantation. Soderwall also showed that excess estrogen could cause failure of the pregnancy at any point, from failure of the embryo to implant, to resorption of the fetus at a late stage of pregnancy."

Now if we look at the female endometrium, which is fed nutrients and oxygen by the spiral arteries, we can see that this environment needs to be kept suitable for the embryo to implant at the eight to ten day mark.[2] There are of course many things that act on the endometrium, one of the biggest offenders being estrogen.

> *"Estrogen acting alone or with insufficient progesterone causes spasms in the spiral arteries that provide oxygen and nutrients to the endometrium. This seems to be the basis for menstruation, and is also believed to be a factor in miscarriage."*
>
> - Ray Peat, PhD.

If we investigate this mechanism a bit more, we will see that estrogen creates the scenario above for many reasons:

1. Estrogen, along with unsaturated fats, wastes Vitamin E. Vitamin E is anti-estrogenic. Vitamin E and progesterone ensure the tissues and the embryo adequate oxygen and nutrients. Estrogen pulls oxygen and nutrients away from tissues and organs, thus creating "suffocation."
2. Excess estrogen or progesterone deficiency consumes oxygen at a high rate, lowering oxygen concentrations. *"Aged tissue has a diminished respiratory capacity."* - Ray Peat, PhD
3. High levels of estrogen or low levels of progesterone have a profound effect on the ovaries. P.M. Wise showed that estrogen inhibits cells that shut off the pituitary gonadotrophins FSH and LH. High levels of FSH and LH disturb the ovaries and lower progesterone levels. However, too much progesterone will decrease FSH and LH.

---

[2] From our standpoint, implantation happens around day 6, and can occur til around day 10. There is some variance based on different peoples work. But the environment does play a huge role.
(http://raypeat.com/articles/articles/menopause.shtml)

4. Histamine mimics estrogen's actions on the uterus, and anti-histamines, such as salt and coconut oil, will block estrogen's effects.
5. Estrogen excess with a Vitamin E deficiency intensifies the formation of age pigment called lipofuscin. Unsaturated fats + iron + estrogen = lipofuscin. Estrogen is a powerful stimulant of iron absorption, and iron is involved in peroxidation that produces age pigment. Lipofuscin and estrogen consume both oxygen and fuel at a high rate with no usable cellular energy on the return. It has been shown by Gritx and Rahko that a diet high in unsaturated fats and deficient in Vitamin E contributes to lipofuscin or age pigment.
    a. Lipofuscin contains a heme group that produces carbon monoxide, a respiratory poison that interferes with cellular respiration by wasting oxygen.
    b. A cell's basic mechanism of adaptation is the production of new proteins and the destruction of old proteins. Lipofuscin directly inhibits the proteolytic enzymes that break down proteins. Unsaturated fats have a similar action. Both lead to free radical production.
6. Estrogen and unsaturated fats suppress thyroid hormone. Adequate thyroid hormone provides optimal cellular respiration and the effective use of oxygen and carbon dioxide production. Low thyroid allows estrogen to accumulate in the tissues whereas thyroid hormone facilitates the elimination of estrogen and produces the protective progesterone.
7. Hans Selye, MD, showed that estrogen alone mimics the shock phase of the stress reaction. He pointed out that estrogen causes the pituitary to secrete prolactin and ACTH. Both of these hormones cause the ovaries to stop producing progesterone and contribute to aging, atrophy, and infertility.

> *ACTH will stimulate the production of cortisol, pushing the body deeper into a catabolic survival state. The body is thinking about safety and security, not reproduction.*
>
> *"Stress lowers progesterone and a deficiency will prevent implantation and result in anovulatory cycles."*
>
> - Ray Peat, PhD

8. Estrogen has been qualified as a female hormone. For this reason, menopausal infertility has been identified as an estrogen deficiency. This is dangerous thinking. To begin with, estrogen is not a female hormone; both men and women produce it in the adrenals and the breast tissue. Women also produce estrogen in the fat cells and the ovaries. More weight gain leads to excess estrogen. Progesterone, on the other hand, can only be produced by the corpora lutea in the ovaries. In states of chronic stress or hypometabolism, progesterone production is inhibited by cortisol, leading to deficiencies in progesterone. Progesterone is a pro-gestational hormone. Without adequate amounts to oppose estrogen, "suffocation" will occur within the uterus, leading to infertility issues and miscarriages eight to ten weeks following conception.

In conclusion, excess estrogen and unsaturated fats damage the cell's ability to breathe, which leads to high rates of oxygen consumption. Conception cannot occur when oxygen is being consumed at high rates, as it leaves no viable oxygen left for the embryo.

Restoring fertility processes and function may require a look into the functionality of the metabolism in its wholeness, which we will explore in the second part of this book.

Menopause

> *"Between the ages of 50 and 55, about 60% of women experience episodes of flushing and sweating. Around the same age, late 40s to mid-50s, men being to have sudden increase of some of the same health problems, including night sweats, anxiety, and insomnia."*
>
> - Ray Peat, PhD

Hot flashes have always been associated with menopause, which, according to Ray Peat, is a major sign of aging. What has come to our attention and a fact in need of real consideration is the presence of symptoms of menopause being found not only in menopausal women but women much younger—in their 20s and 30s. In today's society, even men are being plagued by menopausal-like hot flashes!

There is no such thing as a male hormone and a female hormone. All human bodies produce ALL the steroidal hormones (estrogen, progesterone, testosterone, DHEA, pregnenolone) with the only difference being how much. How much is dependent not only on sex, which is primary, but many other internal and external factors. Hot flashes are a symptom of hormonal metabolic dysfunction in both men and women. Though this book is focused on female health, this consideration can be applied to both men and women, young and old.

What exactly is a hot flash? A hot flash has nothing to do with outdoor/indoor temperatures or global warming. Hot flashes are a symptom of increased vasodilation of the blood vessels. Increased vasodilation causes increased heat loss through the skin and a decrease in heat production internally and at the cellular level. Any decline in heat production causes a decrease in energy production and body temperature.

In relation to the production of steroidal hormones, estrogen, serotonin, tryptophan, and melatonin are all hypothermic in nature. This means they all contribute to the process that causes hot flashes. This topic is very extensive so we will not be touching on it directly. We will instead be focusing here on our old "friend," estrogen.

The "female" hormone estrogen is a popular hormone replacement commonly prescribed by medical doctors to assist with hormonal imbalances. It is a popular belief that estrogen causes the blood vessels to relax and dilate, making it useful in protecting against hot flashes. (Thus improving dilation, improving circulation, and protecting against hypertension.)

What is so interesting is the fact that there are repeated studies on the toxicity of excess estrogen caused internally and/or through external supplementation. Estrogen *causes* increased vasodilation of the blood vessels, increased blood pressure, up-regulation of inflammatory hormones, and suppression of the thyroid and other energy-building systems in the body. Estrogen is a major contributor to almost all degenerative diseases. Estrogen is produced in many places in the body and is heavily influenced by environmental factors.

> *"Estrogen makes the toxic mediator producing cells in the liver (Kupffer cells) 15x more sensitive to LPS (endotoxin). This increases the alarm responses and activation of inflammatory mediators; phospholipases, nitric oxide synthase, tumor necrosis factor (TNF), interleukins and the enzymes that form prostaglandins from polyunsaturated fatty acids."*
>
> - The Metabolic Blueprint: Design of the GI System

Nitric oxide (NO) is increased in women going through menopause (Watanabe, et al., 2000), and is also increased by inflammation. Inhibitors of NO reduce vasodilation during hot flashes (Hubing, et al., 2010). Endotoxin or LPS has been show to increase NO, and estrogen has been shown to increase LPS. "Plasma nitrite levels and inducible nitric oxide synthase in the liver were also elevated significantly in estrogen-treated rats 6 h after LPS." According to Ray Peat, PhD, consuming foods with Vitamin B12 and Vitamin E are antidotal to NO. Cascara Sagrada has also been shown to inhibit the formation of NO and fatty acid synthesis.

> *"Estrogen increases the free fatty acids (FFA) circulating in the blood."*
> - Ray Peat PhD

FFAs in the blood from polyunsaturated fats shift oxidative metabolism away from glucose oxidation and towards lipid oxidation. This lowers oxidative energy production, thyroid production, and body temperature, and leads to hibernated sleep or torpor (poor quality rest).

It is very rare that women will ever need to supplement with estrogen. In fact, Ray Peat, PhD, explains, "There is no evidence that women experiencing hot flashes were deficient in estrogen (in fact, there was evidence that they weren't), and there was evidence that hot flashes began when the first menstrual period was missed, which coincided with, and resulted from, a failure to produce function corpus luteum, preventing the production of a normal amount of progesterone."

According to Ray Peat, PhD, one of the things progesterone does is stabilize blood sugar. "In one experiment, hot flashes were found to be increased by lowering blood sugar, and decreased by moderately increasing blood sugar (Dormire and Reame, 2003)." It has been shown as well that a decrease in progesterone will increase the production of NO.

Is Estrogen Supplementation an Appropriate Approach?

Most women are encouraged to take estrogen to decrease hot flashes. In some women, it does work, and in the other half, it doesn't. Based on our own research and working with women, we believe that the oxidative state of the individual taking the estrogen is the real issue. In women who are severely hypothyroid and have low body temperature, taking the estrogen lowers their core temperature even more, thus pushing them deeper into their already anti-metabolic state and reducing flushes. According to Ray Peat, PhD, "Menopause itself is the result of prolonged exposure to estrogen; very large doses of estrogen can, in many women, stop the flushing."

On the flip side, this must be questioned. The simple fact that estrogen lowers body temperature clues us in to the effects this approach may be having on a deeper cellular level. It might even be suggested that this reduction in hot flashes influenced by estrogen supplementation symbolizes the current state of hormonal imbalance.

Estrogen and the Nervous System

The nervous system is extremely sensitive to the effects of estrogen. Hypoglycemia by way of the adrenal cortex will increase estrogen, which increases hot flashes. Estrogen alone will stimulate the adrenal cortex and increase cortisol. According to Ray Peat, PhD, "CRH causes vasodilation and is more active in the presence of estrogen."

Through this process, the increased production of cortisol will have many physiologic affects. In relation to hot flashes, cortisol:

– Increases protein turnover
– Increases overall heat production
– Stimulates adrenaline, which increases vasodilation

In conclusion, regulating the metabolism through blood sugar stabilization will inhibit estrogen production, inhibit cortisol production, increase thyroid production, normalize body temperature…and eliminate hot flashes! We'll take a look at metabolism and blood sugar in the next chapter.

Metabolism

In this and the following chapters, we're going to take a look at the best ways for you to balance your hormones and achieve overall health. We'll start with the very basics, your metabolism. Without the solid foundation of metabolic health, other steps will not be as successful and may fail altogether. Once you learn to assess your metabolic health, you'll learn to support your body with good nutrition. Then we'll move on to lifestyle factors—sleep, stress, exercise, and detoxification. Let's get started!

We know that the word "metabolism" automatically gets you thinking about diets and losing weight. While those are related, metabolism is so much more than that. In this section of the book, you'll learn about your metabolism, how it affects your health, and easy ways to determine your own metabolic health. While healing your metabolism is not the only factor in your health blueprint, it plays such a large role. Because of that, you may find that many symptoms decrease in severity or go away altogether when you get this part of your health routine in place.

Metabolism is a term that refers to all the biochemical reactions that occur within the cells of the human body. These reactions are designed to keep the cells functioning and, more important, are essential to maintaining the living state of the body. How your cells are breathing and producing energy—not how skinny you are or how much you work out—dictates health.

Nutrition is the key to metabolism. The carbohydrates, proteins, and fats we consume contain essential nutrients (calories and necessary chemicals) that the body cannot synthesize itself. Food provides the substances essential for the building, upkeep, and repair of body tissues and for the efficient functioning of the body. We'll take a look at nutrition in the following chapter. For now, let's look at a few ways to determine the state of your metabolic health.

Assessing the state of your metabolism provides extremely useful information when working to restore energy production in the body. Understanding how your cells are breathing clues you in to how each system is functioning, which allows you to define the most appropriate resources for healing to occur from the inside-out vs. the outside-in.

There are many inexpensive and highly effective ways to monitor metabolic efficiency and to stay in tune with how your body is responding to the changes you will be making. Let's take a look at some of these simple and low-cost tools now.

Body Temperature and Pulse

Measuring basal body temperature and pulse provides you with information about the strength of your metabolic function and how efficiently you may or may not be producing energy/heat in your body. Normal body temperature can range from 97.8 - 98.6 F (36.6 - 37.0 C). A normal pattern will be lower temps in the morning, a peak mid-day, and decline again in the evening.

The pulse can be measured in the amount of times your heart beats per minute. When the metabolism is strong, the pulse will be strong; when the metabolism is weak, the pulse too will be weak. The more normal it is, the more efficiently nutrients and oxygen are being delivered to the cells.

Recording your temperature and pulse allows you to:

- Assess hormonal fluctuation influenced by the body's ability to meet daily demands

- Identify subclinical hypothyroidism
- Identify adrenal and blood sugar influences on metabolism

When body temperature and pulses are out of normal range, it indicates a stress on the system. Stress on the system stimulates a slew of inflammatory hormones, such as adrenaline, cortisol, prolactin, estrogen, serotonin, etc., all of which create suppression and inhibition of the production of energy and much more.

Low body temperature:

- Disrupts digestive function, leading to the inability to break down and absorb nutrients- (malnourishment)
- Suppresses thyroid function
- Inhibits the production of protective steroidal hormones
- Creates mineral imbalances
- Wastes oxygen, leading to lactic acid production, inhibiting glycogen storage, and rapidly wasting stored energy
- Leads to a breakdown in muscle tissue
- Forces an adrenaline compensation

The more you can regulate blood sugar and provide the body what it needs, the less these things will occur. Over time, consistency in nutrition and lifestyle will restore energy metabolism, increase energy in the body, and increase overall health!

3 Ways to Measure Body Temperature:

1. **Axillary:** Suggested by Broda Barnes as most accurate upon waking in the morning, while the body is in a restful state.
2. **Oral:** Chronic sinus issues are associated with hypometabolism (hypothyroidism) and can raise oral temperatures by almost one degree.
3. **Rectal**

Whatever method you choose, stay consistent to avoid extreme variations. Normal fluctuations do occur during the course of a woman's menstrual cycle, however. Because of this:

- Menstruating women should take their temperature on the 2nd and 3rd day of their menstrual cycle.
- Young girls, women with irregular cycles, and post-menopausal women can take it any time of the month.

<u>**How to Measure Your Pulse:**</u>

* Use your fingers when taking your pulse and avoid using your thumb as it has its own pulse.

Measuring your radial pulse (inside of wrist):

- Place the pads of your index and middle finger just below the wrist crease at the base of the thumb. Press lightly until you feel a pulse.

Measuring the carotid pulse (side of neck):

- Place the pads of your index and middle finger about halfway between your ear and your chin right at the base of the jawbone. Press lightly until you feel a pulse.
- Using a watch or a clock with a second hand, count the number of beats per minute.

Best times to take temperature and pulse:

- Upon waking in bed, prior to sitting up. Your waking pulse and temperature are your baseline.
- 20 min after breakfast, lunch, and dinner.
- Prior to going to bed.

Commit to logging your temperature and pulse three days of each week. Take the other four days of the week off and simply continue implementing the balance, ratio, and frequency of your meals and lifestyle adjustments that we'll discuss in later chapters.

Common patterns and variations in temp/pulse readings:

- Body temperature ranging between 97.8-98.6F (37C) means your ability to produce energy is efficient and the body is not in a compensatory pattern of energy conversion. Anything below may indicate otherwise.
- Your morning temperature and pulse is your baseline metabolic health.
- After breakfast, your temperature and pulse should increase and remain constant with a slight increase throughout the day. If they drop or do not go up, this is a sign of blood sugar instability. Remember that you are healing and this takes time. You might not hit 98F right away, but as long as you see a steady increase, that is the key.
- Optimal pulse is within a range of 75-85 bpm at rest. Having a low pulse is a sign of thyroid and/or adrenal deficiency. If you notice your pulse is running low, give it some time as this takes a while to normalize.
- Inconsistent fluctuations in body temp and pulse throughout the day despite efforts to manage blood sugar through proper nutrition indicates an adrenal deficiency.
- A high pulse above 85bpm can be a sign of high adrenaline or cortisol.
- Exercise will increase your body temperature and pulse and keep them elevated for an extended period of time. Give yourself a minimum of 30 minutes to recover and normalize post-exercise before taking readings.

Achilles Reflex

How to Measure:

- Kneel on a chair with your foot dangling off the chair. Tap the Achilles tendon directly with a reflex hammer, book, etc. As you tap the tendon, the foot should plantar flex briskly without delay.

Results: Normal is when there is a brisk reflex and return bilaterally. A delayed response could be an indication of low thyroid.

Under-Shirt Test

How to Measure:

- Place your hands on your bare skin below your shirt. If your hands are cold on your skin, something in the environment (food choices, balance, lifestyle) is interfering with energy production.

Temperature of Hands, Feet, and Nose

- Cold hands and feet indicate increased adrenaline, low pulse, and low body temperature
- Cold nose typically means low stored glycogen in the liver

Blood Pressure Differential

- In a perfect world, ideal BP is 120/80. If you feel your BP is above these numbers, we recommend talking to your MD.
- For this test, calculate your BP. The differential is the difference between both numbers. If your differential is 50 or lower, this means your heart is working efficiently.

Our Thoughts on Lab Testing

Lab testing has become a very common practice among alternative health care practitioners. Labs can be helpful in providing information about different systems in the body, but the problem with labs and how they are being used is:

- They are being used as diagnostic tools
- Practitioners are treating labs instead of the human being in front of them.
- Any breakdown in the system is either the cause OR effect of something greater occurring. Labs can identify this but cannot determine what the root cause is, potentially leaving the issue unresolved even following treatment.
- Labs are expensive and they are often accompanied by a supplement protocol that is more cost with little return.

Food & Nutrition

Now that you have some idea of the problems associated with a low metabolism and how to evaluate the state of your metabolism, you're probably wondering what, if anything, you can do to fix it. Don't worry—this isn't the part where we tell you that you need drugs or even supplements. Much of the healing that can occur comes through simple everyday practices. The practice that provides the biggest bang for your buck is food.

What you eat and how you eat it is the basis of healing. But food, as you probably already know, can also harm. So how can you tell the difference? With all the diet plans out there, how do you really know what to eat?

What to Eat

Have you ever noticed that most diets promoted by diet gurus and nutrition "experts" usually involve eliminating or severely restricting a specific food group? Paleo or low-carb dieters seek to limit carbohydrate intake. Vegans and vegetarians often limit protein as a matter of course. And back in the 90s, low-fat diets were all the rage (and, in fact, are still promoted by major medical associations for heart health despite the overwhelming evidence to the contrary—we need fat for good health!).

Well, we're here to give you some good news. Everyone needs *all three* macronutrients—fats, carbohydrates, and protein—to promote good health and, especially, to help heal a broken metabolism and to balance hormones. To give you an idea of why these three macros are so essential to health, let's break them down now.

Fatty acids are found in every cell in the body and are essential to human survival. Fats:

- Are required for growth and development.
- Support satiation and help slow the digestion of carbohydrates and proteins.
- Are really important when it comes to cravings!
- Are essential for proper functioning of the nerves and the brain.
- Are used as a back-up energy source. This is why the body converts excess sugar into fat when you don't eat enough fat.
- Assist in the absorption and transportation of vitamins A, D, E, and K through the bloodstream to where they are needed.
- Act as an antioxidant and protect the cells.

Saturated fatty acids interact the least with other molecules in the body and provide the most stable structure. Polyunsaturated fatty acids (PUFA's) are much more interactive and susceptible to oxidation in human tissues. These oxidative processes damage enzymes and energy production at the cellular level.

Because of this, we recommend getting most of your fats as saturated fats (coconut oil, heavy cream, animal tallow, butter), some as monounsaturated (olive oil and avocados), and eliminating PUFA's (found in safflower, sunflower, corn, soybean, cottonseed, peanut, canola, and other "vegetable" oils) as much as possible.

Proteins make up approximately 40% of the body's weight and serve in:

- Repair, replacement, and regeneration of every tissue and cell in the body.

- Liver support and function. This is essential to helping your body detoxify excess estrogen.
- The production of hormones and enzymes such as thyroid. Enzymes are essential to digestion and support in energy production.

Most of your protein calories should come from power proteins, such as broth, gelatin, dairy, eggs, fish, shellfish, and liver (1x/week). Most plant proteins are incomplete and can interfere with the metabolic process.

When carbohydrates are in the proper balance and accompanied by proteins and fats:

- The tissues and cells of the body are provided their primary and preferred source of energy.
- The central nervous system, kidneys, brain, and muscles (including the heart) are properly nourished. Did you know glucose is the only fuel used by brain cells? Neurons cannot store glucose; they depend on the bloodstream to deliver a constant supply of this precious fuel!
- They act similarly to time-released capsules of sugar. Carbohydrates, in the form of glycogen (energy), are stored in the liver and muscles for back-up energy throughout the day.
- They enhance digestive function, keeping things moving along while ensuring the proper breakdown and absorption of nutrients.
- They assist in the conversion of inactive thyroid hormone (T4) into active thyroid hormone (T3), the master of metabolism. Up to 80% of thyroid is converted in the liver. This conversion requires glucose from carbohydrates!

We recommend eliminating all grains, breads, and pastas…even if gluten-free. Carbohydrates such as root vegetables and squashes are preferred starches over grains and potatoes. These starches contain both fructose and glucose and are loaded with anti-fungal properties, which can be beneficial in the absorption of toxins and other bacteria in the intestines (endotoxin, estrogen). Fruit is also an acceptable source of carbs.

How to Eat

How you eat is nearly as important as what you eat.

Eat frequent small meals throughout the day, each containing a balance of macronutrients. All three macronutrients in balance are equally important for managing blood glucose and providing lasting energy. Eliminating any one of the three macronutrients from a snack or a meal can easily inhibit energy production. Managing blood glucose is one of the best ways to support hormone balance in the body.

As a starting point, begin using a balance of 50% carbohydrates, 25% protein, and 25% fat. For those who are very aware of how sensitive they are to sugar, reducing the carbs to 40% and increasing the protein and fats to 30% might be a better option. Although the right types of sugars are essential to health, when the body is healing, it is still very reactive. Too much sugar can challenge one's ability to manage blood glucose and keep the body highly activated. Start slowly and never without a baseline! If you find yourself with food cravings or you are very hungry soon after a meal, take a mental note of this. You may need more food or a better balance.

As you move forward, you will learn what ratios work best for you. For now, just be sure each time you eat to take a moment and identify your carbohydrates, proteins, and fats. Visually pie-charting your plate can be very helpful in identifying a good balance.

One of the most important factors in healing is consistency and creating rhythms in your life. The human body is very similar to that of a child with a schedule versus a child without. When the body knows what is coming next, it is calm, balanced, settled, and able to respond to life as it comes. When the body is not receiving what it needs, it is in internal chaos, which leads to extreme hormonal fluctuations throughout the day, cravings, depression, frustration, irritability, fatigue, headaches, allergies, foggy thinking, dizziness, and so much more.

Infrequent eating creates a deficiency in energy, contributing to rapid and frequent fluctuations in blood sugar throughout the day, which easily translates into restless nights and very often waking up between 1 a.m. and 3 a.m., making it very difficult to get back to sleep.

Eating small meals throughout the day provides the body with what it needs to meet the demands of life. This supports and helps to normalize blood sugar and reduces the stress load on the system, all while re-teaching your body how to store glycogen!

Eating frequent, balanced meals throughout the day increase energy, keeps your nervous system calm, and keeps you much happier. Over time, hormonal cycles will restore themselves, you will get the rest you need, and you will wake up refreshed and ready to meet the day.

Take notice of how a meal makes you feel. Does it warm your body? Does it make you tired, cold, or irritable? Does it give you energy and help you focus? Are you hungry soon after a meal? The more awareness you have, the better you will be at identifying your personal tools.

Food Logging

Food logging provides purpose, growth, and opportunity to create a "diet" and lifestyle more suitable for you. Yes, logging takes some getting used to, which is why we highly recommend starting slowly, but as you become more acquainted with it, you'll find that it becomes easier.

The only way to know what nutrition and lifestyle changes you need to make is to observe what exactly is creating stress in your body. We know that when metabolism is less than optimal, the body must compensate, and in doing so, it secretes high amounts of excitatory hormones. Over time, we adapt to these excitable states and can no longer recognize the signals of stress.

Hans Selye observed in those habituated to high levels of internal stress since early childhood that it is the absence of stress that creates unease. Very common today is the addiction to stress hormones, as the very absence of them can evoke boredom and a sense of meaninglessness. For others, stress is related to areas of work, family, relationships, finances, or health. Sensations of agitation, irritability, and the like do not always define stress, nor are they necessarily perceived when people are stressed.

In short, Selye explains, stress is not a matter of subjective feeling, but a measure of objective physiological events in the body involving the brain, endocrine system, immune system, and other organs.

Logging provides a degree of objective measures that create awareness and an opportunity to understand your body and the messages it is sending.

Food logging serves a couple of really important purposes:

1. It allows you to begin to see how your body is in relationship with the world around you (e.g., nutrition, lifestyle, emotions, exercise). Remember, many of us no longer can identify what stress FEELS like in the body.
2. Logging paints the picture and provides all the information you need to begin making the proper modifications. This chapter is designed to help you create a nutrition plan that supports your metabolic function, which in turn helps every level of your health.
3. It helps you begin to see what balanced nutrients look like on a plate. Familiarizing yourself with what balance and portions work for you frees you to enjoy your life. You are no longer a prisoner, not knowing what to eat or living in fear of how you might feel after.
4. Everyone has their own definition of health and we encourage you to define yours. Why is getting healthy important to you? Exploring these ideas will help you to discover a source of motivation.

Stress

Healing the body is impossible when the body is in a state of stress. Elevated stress hormones suppress and inhibit many supportive functions in the body and lead to deficiencies in the vitamins and minerals needed as catalysts for these functions. Remember how stress can throw the estrogen-progesterone ratio out of balance? Managing stress is a key step in balancing hormonal health.

Take a moment here and there throughout the day to check in with yourself and notice how you are feeling in your body. There is so much chatter in our lives, along with a lot of influences on how we should be feeling, doing, thinking, looking, etc. All this noise has interfered with our innate ability to identify what we need for ourselves by what our body is communicating.

Take this as an opportunity to come back into relationship with what your body is communicating. As we dive deeper into fine-tuning, you will begin to be able to correlate what is going on in your life with how your body is behaving in response to your environment. This is vital information for you in creating a life of health and vitality.

Unfortunately, many of us live in a constant state of stress and are often unable to recognize when this unnatural state has taken over as the new normal. Do any of the following symptoms of a chronic stress state sound familiar to you?

What Adrenaline Looks and Feels Like:

- Cravings
- Allergies
- Headaches
- Bad dreams and/or nightmares
- Binge eating
- Nervous stomach, cramps
- Poor concentration
- Insomnia
- Irritability
- Sleepiness
- Indecision
- Depression
- Dizziness, lightheadedness
- Nervous eating
- Heart palpitations
- Tremors

So You're Stressed…Now What?

1. **Balance blood sugar.** Include all three macronutrients at each meal and eating at regular intervals.
2. **Avoid unsaturated fats.** Elevated estrogen levels perpetuate chronic stress and deplete glycogen storages in the liver. This combination provokes the release of fatty acids into the bloodstream to be converted into glucose and used as energy. PUFA's inhibit cellular respiration, pushing the body deeper into the vicious cycle of inflammation. All of this equals STRESS!
3. **Take frequent Epsom salt baths.** Besides being relaxing, they're also a great detoxifier. Excess estrogen leads to water retention secondary to increased uptake of water in the tissues and low albumin levels in the liver caused by malnutrition and over-burdening of the liver. Estrogen dominance leads to an excessive uptake of magnesium, creating an imbalance in intra- and extracellular minerals. This can lead to water retention due to the uptake of sodium into the cell secondary to magnesium deficiency.
4. **Get adequate sleep** (see chapter on Sleep).

5. **Avoid over-exercising** (see chapter on Exercise).
6. **Practice deep breathing.** Meditation, yoga, tai chi, and other mindfulness practices have also proven very successful in managing stress.

Remember, your body doesn't know if you're being chased by a lion or are simply late for a meeting at work—the damage to your health is the same.

Decoding Cravings

Have you ever noticed how food cravings often parallel times of stress and anxiety? Well, guess what, this is no mistake! Cravings go way beyond the simple need to appease hunger. Rather, they are a confounding cocktail of body, brain, and chemicals packed with enormous amounts of power.

The body is constantly and forever working to maintain a state of balance, and in doing so, it communicates very clear messages to us throughout each day. It informs us when it is time to rest, when we are thirsty, when we are hungry or too full, when we need to eliminate, and when there is excess stress (constipation, insomnia, fatigue, lack of focus, nausea, suppressed appetite). Food cravings are a clear signal from the body that the energy being received is not adequate to the demands needing to be fulfilled.

Cravings are also a clear-cut signal that blood sugar is not being managed, and managing blood sugar is a key to balancing hormones.

When blood sugar is either too high or too low, the cells are not receiving what they require to produce energy. Glucose is the cells' best friend and is essential to energy production. Any time the body falls below a normal blood glucose level, adrenaline and cortisol are released as a signal to release stored glycogen. If the body does not receive enough dietary carbohydrates or the glycogen storage sites are empty, the body has an adaptive survival response. ("Adaptive" meaning that the body has a backup, alternative energy-producing mechanism because it understands how essential sugar is to our survival.) Although a very common pattern being witnessed in our society, this adapted state is not a state we should be sustaining life in and contributes greatly to cravings!

Daily Choices Create Cravings

Everything we come up against in our day has the potential to influence cravings when the body is not being supported in the appropriate way. There are several hormones involved in the process, so the more balance we can define in life, the fewer cravings and the more energy we will have! Here are some of the top sources of cravings:

1. Poor Food Choices

<u>Relying on plants for proteins.</u> Many people believe they can receive complete protein through the consumption of grains, lentils, soy, and beans and no animal protein. This might be partially true in the proper combination but never without sacrifice to the needs of the human body. Grains, lentils, soy, and beans tend to be low-quality nutrients and contain PUFA's, which can inhibit energy production in the body.

These "protein" sources:

- Lower protein digestion
- Inhibit mineral (such as calcium and zinc) absorption
- Lower oxygen input to your cells = decreased energy production Contain phytoestrogens, which increase estrogen = edema, increase in cortisol, blood sugar dysregulation, and much more

<u>**Processed foods**</u> - also referred to as non-foods, they contain loads of preservatives, have no nutritional value, and actually take more energy to break down than they offer in return. Low energy coincides with some degree of malnourishment. Our nutrients are essential to every function in our body. Eating processed foods is a waste of time and money.

***There are going to be times when we are just not prepared and have nothing to eat. Do the very best you can in what you have to choose from. Eating always takes priority!

2. Eating out of balance. Too much protein, not enough carbohydrate, and vice versa both contribute to blood sugar dysregulation. Keep meals balanced and frequent = normalize blood sugar = stabilize hormones = decrease inflammation = increase absorption and nourishment = healthier metabolism = ENERGY!!!

3. Diet deficient in protein. Consuming high-quality, non-inflammatory protein plays an essential role in human physiology. Protein is digested in the stomach, absorbed in the small intestine, and is transported to the liver where it supports the production of thyroid hormone and estrogen detoxification. Diets deficient in protein, due to either low consumption or malabsorption, increase circulating estrogen and decrease thyroid hormone production, both of which block energy production.

When protein is insufficient, the body will compensate by eating itself. Not a good scenario! Whether you are eating muscle meats or your body is eating itself, when inflammation is underlying, this metabolism of amino acids can cause the body to become highly excitable. Cortisol is the catalyst to this catabolic conundrum and leads to issues managing blood sugar, inhibition of thyroid hormone production, and burdening of the liver.

4. Limiting or avoiding optimal carbohydrates in the diet. Carbohydrates dominate energy production and are the human body's primary and preferred source of fuel. Without this essential macronutrient, the body is forced into an adaptive survival state, which stresses the physiology and leads to rapid degeneration and chronic fatigue.

5. Poor food frequency: As the body adapts into alternative energy production, it decreases O2 consumption. Low levels of O2 interrupt cellular respiration and shifting the cells' energy production away from CO2 and towards the production of lactic acid. Lactic acid causes the liver to waste glucose. This coupled with low carbohydrate diets is a recipe for disaster.

By eating frequent balanced meals, you are giving the body what it needs, reducing the burden on the system, reducing inflammatory cycles, increasing oxygen consumption and CO_2 production, and restoring metabolic health in the body!

6. Poor food ratios: This is complex and takes awareness, time, and consistency of logging to figure out. But the more we pay attention to what is working for us based on body temperature and pulse, the more we align our nutrition to our physiology.

7. Over-training: The exercise of today is much different than the exercise of our ancestors. Our ancestors, for one, had a much higher exposure to sunlight and less exposure to dioxins, estrogen, mercury, fluoride, radiation, and PUFA's. These are all anti-metabolic stressors, and when coupled with too much of the wrong exercise and not enough of the correct exercise, they induce an aging effect. In this day and age, most are in a hypo-metabolic state, and this combination is posing a huge threat to our health.

Most people, including health professionals, view weight gain as a symptom of too little activity and think that increasing exercise frequency (with very little thought into exercise variables) is the most logical path to success. Dianna Schwarzbien, MD, states that you must get healthy to lose weight, not lose weight to get healthy!

Excess weight is a sign of a disrupted metabolism. Is exercise important? Absolutely! We are designed to move. HOW we move and, even more importantly, how we are supporting our energy needs around our movement is of primary importance.

In our experience, most people are eating WAY TOO FEW calories are in full-on survival mode, and exercise is doing nothing but making it all worse!

8. Environmental toxins (see chapter on Detoxification).

9. Lack of sleep (see chapter on Sleep).

10. Emotional Stress: This can be a little tricky and is not the focus of this book, but we do acknowledge that it is a huge piece to the healing puzzle. Greatest take away is that a stress is a stress is a stress! Stress affects how our body uses energy and challenges our ability to maintain homeostasis.

How emotional stress can be supported:

- Study the work of JP Sears:
  www.innerawakeningsonline.com
- Study the work of John McMullin:
  www.journeysofwisdom.com
- Practice daily qi gong, tai chi, or meditation
- Discover or reconnect with a hobby
- Change how you view, perceive, and react to certain situations in your life. Energy follows intent! What do you want to put energy into?

11. Not meeting your metabolic demands: Calories are the most important part of meeting your demands. Most people under-eat! When healing, the body requires more energy in order to regulate, heal the body, and create energy. Not getting enough calories pushes your body into survival mode. The amount of calories you need will vary per day, per week, or per season depending on menstrual cycles, stressors in your life, and the healing phase you are in.

12. Eating too much too fast: We can't say this enough…slow down, embrace what you are doing, and enjoy the journey! This takes time, so patience is key. Going too fast and eating too much too soon will be too much stress for the body. The most common ways the body expresses this is through your symptoms getting worse, slow progress, and weight gain.

Take the time to chew your food, sip your drinks, sit down when eating, and take time out to enjoy the food you are ingesting! Honor your body!

Who Craves Salt?

Anyone familiar with salt cravings? Just another way your body is communicating its needs. Paying attention to this signal can really pay off in the end!

Sodium is essential both physiologically and biochemically in keeping the body balanced. When the body is in a hypo-metabolic state, it loses sodium in the urine, which triggers adrenaline production.

The addition of salt in the right amounts can aid in:

- Normalizing blood pressure
- Increasing circulatory efficiency
- Reducing edema
- Down-regulating aldosterone and adrenaline, and improving sleep

Salting your foods to taste is all you need. Start with a small amount each day and work up to what works for you. Morton's pickling salt or a white Celtic sea salt are preferred sources.

Curb the Cravings Snack Ideas

Liquid Energy:

***These three can be turned into popsicles!

1. Orange Creamsicle - OJ, cream or coconut milk, gelatin, salt
2. Fruit Smoothie - Frozen fruit, OJ, coconut milk, gelatin
3. Hot Cacao - coconut milk, water, honey, cacao powder, gelatin, salt

Cup of Broth with Cooked Apples - Add a tbsp. of protein and dash of coconut oil

Chicken salad or egg salad with fresh fruit or OJ - Make it your own! We like to add fruit to our salad, include a little goat cheese, and mix it up. If you like it a little more traditional, purchase an olive oil based mayo or make your own!

Mini-Meals - Have a half portion of a meal for snack. It is already made and will give you some more variety.

Sleep

Do you have trouble falling asleep, staying asleep, or waking up? Do you rely on supplements or medical drugs in order to catch a few Z's? There are many things that are thought to cause sleep disturbances, including aging, menopause, eating too much sugar before bed, or eating too close to going to bed. The one thing these all have in common is their direct effect on blood glucose management.

What if all sleep issues came down to regulating blood sugar in order to down-regulate inflammatory markers like serotonin, aldosterone, cortisol, adrenaline, prolactin, estrogen, and melatonin?

Our sleep period is a time of fasting, which creates instabilities in blood sugar. This can pose a real problem for those in an adrenaline compensation or hypo-metabolic state to begin with. Under this adaptive survival mechanism, the body is unable to store adequate glycogen to support the need while at rest, amplifying the hormonal response. Waking between 2 and 4 a.m. with elevated heart rate and anxiety and being unable to get back to sleep is a sign this is happening.

The most common reason people are unable to fall asleep or stay asleep is the inability to regulate their metabolism during both the day and night. The thyroid regulates metabolism, which is correlated with overall body temperature. In a hypo-metabolic state, there is an adaptive increase in the sympathetic nervous system, which produces more adrenaline. The adrenaline helps to sustain blood sugar and body temperature by causing vasoconstriction to the skin (cold hands and feet) but can also lead to disrupted sleep and an accelerated heartbeat. This is common with PMS, menopause, depression, hypothyroidism, and aging.

According to Ray Peat, "Blood sugar falls at night, and the body relies on the glucose stored in the liver as glycogen for energy, and hypothyroid people store very little sugar. As a result, adrenaline and cortisol begin to rise almost as soon as a person goes to bed. In hypothyroid people, they rise very high, with the adrenaline usually peaking around 1 or 2 a.m., and the cortisol peaking around dawn; the high cortisol raises blood sugar as morning approaches and allows adrenaline to decline. Some people wake up during the adrenaline peak with a pounding heart and have trouble getting back to sleep unless they eat something."

"If the night-time stress is very high, the adrenaline will still be high until breakfast, increasing both temperature and pulse rate. The cortisol stimulates the breakdown of muscle tissue and its conversion to energy, so it is thermogenic, for some of the same reasons that food is thermogenic."

The goal is for metabolism to work properly, allowing for optimal cellular respiration throughout the night. Going to bed in a hypo-metabolic state will cause sleep problems.

Top Tips for a Better Night's Sleep:

1. "We should go to bed by 10 p.m. and wake up no earlier than 6 a.m." (Paul Chek, HHP). This is secondary to the diurnal rhythm of all your hormones. Work backwards slowly and get as close to the above times as you can in alignment with your lifestyle. Darkness itself is a stress to your body. Stress hormones naturally increase when the sun goes down. Sleep is the body's way of reducing the stress of darkness. Staying up late by choice or due to insomnia will cause an excess of these stress hormones.

2. Setting the stage for a good night's rest requires the regulation of food ratios and frequencies throughout the day. Work on balancing your blood sugar from the first meal to the last meal of the day. This will help to regulate blood sugar throughout the day, keeping inflammatory hormones low and reducing interference with energy production at night.
3. Avoid bright lights, EMF stress, TV, or any other stressful situations one to two hours prior to bedtime. Try using light therapy right up to bedtime. Light is essential for optimal metabolism and cellular respiration. When the sun goes down (or during periods of darkness), our metabolism starts to slow and stress substances can begin to rise. This is why typically at night you will see a lower body temperature than you would midday. Darkness can damage the energy-producing parts of our cells, the mitochondria, but bright light can restore them.
4. Create a bedtime routine that will help to stimulate the parasympathetic nervous system. Take a shower/bath, snack, stretch, read, listen to relaxing music.
5. Take an Epsom Salt bath prior to bed each night. Magnesium creates relaxation of the muscles, displaces calcium, and assists in blood sugar regulation.
6. Make use of a bedtime snack that is carbohydrate- and salt-loaded. Like salt, sugar is anti-stress, raises metabolism, and raises body temperature. Most fruits contain high levels of magnesium and potassium, and dairy contains calcium, all of which benefits cellular energy production and sleep quality. We recommend a glass of milk with salt and some fruit. The calcium in milk will lower parathyroid hormone, which has been shown to be high with insomnia. Another option would be some fresh pulp-free OJ, gelatin, and salt. Finding the right ratios for YOUR body is key!

> *"Hypothyroidism tends to cause the blood and other body fluids to be deficient in both sodium and glucose. Consuming salty carbohydrate foods momentarily makes up to some extent for the thyroid deficiency."*
>
> - Ray Peat, PhD

7. It is important to use salt during the day, but it is critical to load up on it prior to bed. Salty foods are non-excitatory and increase both T3 and CO2.

- Na regulates intracellular Ca by increasing CO_2 production, thus protecting against cell damage and inflammation
- Na is associated with serum albumin, which is important for regulating blood volume and reducing edema
- Decreased Na loss or intake increases serotonin and adrenaline
- Salty foods assists cells in absorbing sugar, thus up-regulating T3 and Mg
- Sodium lowers several stress mediators such as serotonin, adrenaline, cortisol, and aldosterone
- Sodium helps to regulate blood volume and circulation, thus increasing the delivery of O2 and nutrients, increasing body temperature, and raising the production of carbon dioxide
- Na down-regulates PTH, thus regulating Ca metabolism and leading to a decrease in bone loss at night

8. If you are in a phase where you have cold hands and feet, Ray Peat recommends wearing knit socks and/or a hat to bed.
9. If waking during the night is an issue, sleep with a 4 oz. cup of OJ and salt nearby to sip. Sugar and salt will down-regulate cortisol and adrenaline.
10. Using Progest E (Ray Peat, PhD) at night aids in sleep. Progesterone suspended in Vitamin E is anti-estrogenic,

increases cellular respiration, decreases anxiety, and will increase CO2 levels. Please consult your physician before using!

11. Try eating less meat later in the day (past 3 p.m.). Meat is high in tryptophan, which is a precursor to many stress substances like serotonin and melatonin. These are commonly marketed to improve sleep, but serotonin and melatonin lower metabolism and disrupt sleep. Limiting meats later in the day will minimize the nocturnal production of serotonin and melatonin. Other foods besides meats that are high in tryptophan are egg whites and whey protein; these should also not be eaten later in the day.

    High meat consumption relative to calcium intake (from dairy or eggshells) will disrupt calcium metabolism in the small intestine, thus leading to increased parathyroid hormone production. This is associated with insomnia.

    The use of gelatin or broth, which are high in glycine, later in the day is a much better choice for a protein. Broth and gelatin are void of tryptophan, making them non-inflammatory!

12. Trying using a raw carrot salad or bamboo shoots with your second and fourth meals of the day to reduce endotoxin and estrogen reabsorption. Both of these can cause inflammatory responses in the body. During any type of stress, such as darkness or low blood sugar, endotoxin and estrogen will enter the bloodstream and promote a stress reaction, increasing histamine, estrogen, tumor necrosis factor, serotonin, and cortisol. This will disrupt sleep!

13. Avoid exercise late in the day. The optimal time to exercise is based on our circadian rhythm and is between 10 a.m. and 3 p.m. When healing, this is the most optimal time to exercise. Exercise itself is catabolic and will increase many stressful substances in the body. Exercise

will deplete muscle and liver glycogen, which is used to regulate blood sugar throughout the day and while sleeping. It also promotes hyperventilation, in which we lose excessive amounts of CO_2, which lowers steroidal, reproductive, and thyroid hormones. Choosing the right time to exercise will create the least amount of stress on the body. We find sleep disturbance to be the #1 sign of someone overtraining, working out too intensely, etc. See the Exercise chapter for more information.

14. Make use of Carbon Dioxide Therapies. CO_2 is produced by our cells when they are respiring properly and is an anti-stress substance. Many people with sleep issues hyperventilate and lose CO_2 during the day and night. Eating the right foods, ratios, and frequencies is first in regard to regulating CO_2 production at the cellular level. But other therapies such as bag breathing, Buteyko breathing techniques, drinking carbonated water, and making use of baking soda baths can assist as well in the process of trying to get a good night's sleep.

    According to Leon Chaitow, DO, "Hyperventilation is more common in women. Progesterone stimulates respiration, and in the luteal phase, CO_2 levels drop by an average of 25%. Increased stress can increase ventilation at a time when CO_2 levels are already low."

15. Eliminating PUFA's from your diet will have a profound effect on sleep over time. PUFA's are counterproductive to energy production at the cellular level, decrease CO_2, suppress the immune system, lower body temperature and pulse, negatively affect digestion, promote the production of estrogen, and much more!

16. Avoid taking sleep supplements. One of the most common supplements that people take to help with sleep is melatonin. Unfortunately, melatonin does not improve sleep. Melatonin is synthesized from serotonin and leads to an increase in aldosterone (which will increase blood pressure and vasoconstriction of blood to organs),

involutes the thymus, stimulates cortisol, down-regulates the thyroid, and causes edema. Serotonin increases estrogen and produces melatonin, and both lower metabolic rate. That is why taking melatonin before bed is not a good remedy for sleep problems.

In addition, serotonin induced by stress or hypothyroidism is an important factor in producing the torpor of hibernation and lowering the body temperature. Poor sleep quality can be expected when levels are elevated at night. Most hibernating animals have high levels of serotonin. Hibernation is not a deep wave sleep; it is like being awake!

> *"In hibernating animals, the stress of a declining food supply causes increased serotonin production. In humans and animals that don't hibernate, the stress of winter causes very similar changes. Serotonin lowers temperature by decreasing the metabolic rate. Tryptophan and melatonin are also hypothermic. In the winter, more thyroid is needed to maintain a normal rate of metabolism."*
>
> - Ray Peat, PhD

Exercise

When one is in a hypo-metabolic state (estrogen dominant, thyroid conversion issues, liver dysfunction, etc.), the cells are not respiring properly. Exercise added to this equation exacerbates the hypo-metabolic state by increasing energy demands and blood glucose production in order to fuel the cells during a workout session.

When energy demands are not being met or the body lacks the inability to store or convert glycogen, the body will begin to break itself down (muscle tissue) to provide us with the necessary energy. Again, this is a normal process and a reminder of the intelligence of the human body. The problem is that we leave the gym and step back into our busy lives while we are in a major adrenaline compensation. Appetite is suppressed, we fail to refuel the system adequately, and we drive energy production deeper into dysfunction!

Exercise itself tends to halt the production of T3 (the active thyroid hormone) due to the decrease in blood sugar, increase in FFA in the blood, and the rise of adrenaline and cortisol. Most people can restore their T3 levels following exercise. It is those in a hypo-metabolic state who remain in this decreased metabolic state. Exercise, which is a form of stress, convinces your body that T3 is not needed as an adaptive response to the prolonged stress. Taking your pulse and temperature 30 minutes following exercise will help you identify if this is happening to you.

Exercise Smarter Not Harder

- Start exercising slowly and choose the right form that you feel meets your needs. There are many forms of movement!
- Choose the right frequency of exercise to meet your needs.
- Try to exercise outside and get as much sunlight as you can.
- When exercising, you should feel good and enjoy it from beginning to end. If you feel tired, rest. Your body is speaking to you.
- The type of exercise you choose should prepare you for your daily activities.
- Workouts should be no longer than 60 minutes total with rest programmed between sets and exercises.
- The best time to exercise is between 10 a.m. and 3 p.m. If you can, avoid working out first thing in the morning or late at night.
- When needed, the use of a smoothie or drink to sip on before, during, and after your workout can assist in modulating stress. If you stay on top of your nutritional needs throughout the day, this should not be needed.
- Salt your foods to taste to help regulate adrenaline.
- Make use of Epsom salt baths and/or light therapy on your training days.
- Never work out on an empty stomach. Exercise expends energy and making sure there is enough energy to meet these demands will increase nutrient delivery to the muscles and liver, blunt cortisol production, minimize muscle damage, and set the stage for faster recovery.
- Post workout replenishment is of utmost importance and should be consumed within 30 minutes of working out. Post workout meals should be carbohydrate and salt dominant while including protein and fat to assist in regulating blood sugar, blunting cortisol, increasing the

elimination of metabolic waste, and reducing immune system damage. No meal will negate all the hard work you just put in!

- Monitor the stress of exercise using body temperature and pulse 30 minutes after your session. Optimal would be 97.8-98.6 degrees and a pulse no higher than 85 bpm.

Detoxification

Detoxification helps the body manage exposure to endogenous and exogenous substances. The food we eat, the air we breathe, and the water we drink contain toxic substances that must be processed and eliminated by the human body. Toxins formed within the body are referred to as being endogenous. These toxins are byproducts from normal physiological functions, and the breakdown of hormones and other biochemicals.

Many of these exogenous substances we encounter on a daily basis. These substances cannot be seen, tasted, smelled, or felt. As a society, we really do not know the effects these levels of exposure are having on our health.

Studies by the EPA estimated that in 1994, over 2.2 billion pounds of toxic chemicals were released into the environment in the United States. The estimations increased to over 4.7 billion pounds in 2002. Without a doubt, environmental toxins are leading the race as contributing factors in many of the health challenges being faced by people around the world.

Where will we find these toxic substances?

- Food is highly contaminated with chemicals, like styrene and dioxin, antibiotics, hormones, preservatives, additives, fertilizers, herbicides, and pesticides. Residues of un-

detoxified styrene, dioxin, xylene, and 1,4 – dichlorobenzene are found in 100% of human fat biopsies!
- Xenobiotics: styrene (Styrofoam, plastics, etc.), dioxin (bleached products from diapers, milk cartons, etc.), xylene (exhaust, etc.), pesticides, benzene (gasoline and backing of carpets), PCBs (paints, pesticides, gasoline, etc.), xenoestrogens (pesticides, herbicides, fungicides, plastic wrap, etc.), phthalates (plastics), cyanide (almonds), heavy metals (mercury, lead, cadmium, aluminum, etc.). One group of xenobiotics is made up of environmental estrogens, referred to as xenoestrogens, which mimic animal hormones and act as endocrine system disrupters.
- Air is contaminated with petrochemicals. Auto exhaust contains heavy metals and volatile chemicals (formaldehyde, benzene, toluene, etc.).
- Public water is a man-made chemical liquid. Most municipal water is not detoxified, and chemical substances are added to the water (chlorine, fluoride, etc.). www.shop.friendsofwater.com
- Drugs and medications

Research suggests that many cases of cancer may be caused by a compromised ability to adequately detoxify xenobiotics. Normally, the elimination of xenobiotics is accomplished by their conversion to water-soluble chemicals by enzymes in the liver and other tissues that facilitate their elimination. This is not always the case, however. The fat solubility of exogenous xenobiotics enables them to easily penetrate lipid cell membranes and accumulate in fatty tissues. This increases the load on the detoxification pathways and leads to damage.

What You Can Do to Avoid Toxins

We are heavily exposed to these toxins day in and day out, but we cannot live in a bubble. Awareness is key. The following are great ways to be more proactive in protecting your body:

- Choose healthier, high-quality sources of foods not exposed to herbicides and pesticides.
- Discuss with your spouse and/or MD about alternative contraceptive methods.
- Read labels to eliminate products with fluoride. Fluoride is known to inhibit thyroid hormone production.
- Research ways to either filter water or purchase filtered water without fluoride.
- Substitute plastic Tupperware with glass Pyrex storage containers.
- If you have mercury fillings, when the time is right and you feel the need, talk to a Huggins Holistic Dentist about your options for getting mercury fillings removed.
- Begin substituting your commercial cleaning products for more natural ones. Vinegar and water is a brilliant cleaner. As well, there are tons of natural cleaners on the market. Find one that works for you.
- Replace conventional beauty and hygiene products with organic brands or, better yet, make your own! Coconut oil is an amazing moisturizer, and there are loads of DIY body moisturizers, scrubs, shampoos, and toothpastes online. We've included two facial mask recipes at the end of this chapter.

Symptoms of Toxicity

- Fatigue
- Depression
- Weight problems
- Lethargy
- Muscle Pain
- Joint pain
- Memory Loss
- Headaches
- GI issues
- Poor concentration
- Anxiety
- Arthritis
- Infertility
- Cancer
- Auto-immune diseases
- Nutrient deficiencies... and more!

Organs of Detoxification

There are several organs that contribute to the detoxification process. The primary organ of detoxification is the liver and the second is the intestinal mucosal wall. It is here where toxic substances are converted into nontoxic metabolites.

The Liver

The liver is composed of a number of different cells that work together in accomplishing over 500 different functions in the body. The liver's role in neutralizing and excreting xenobiotics and other potentially toxic compounds is delicately balanced with its immunologic response to bacterial toxins and other macromolecules. The liver is especially important for its role of removing excess estrogens in the body (whether exogenous or endogenous), thus preventing estrogen dominance.

Many of the toxic chemicals that enter the body are fat-soluble, which means they dissolve only in fatty or oily solutions and not in water. This makes them difficult for the body to excrete. Fat-soluble chemicals have a high affinity for fat tissues and cell membranes, which are composed of fatty acids and proteins. The liver filters the blood to remove large toxins, synthesizes and secretes bile full of cholesterol and other fat-soluble toxins, and enzymatically disassembles unwanted chemicals.

The liver's role in detoxification:

- Filtration of the blood: 75% of the liver's blood supply is venous, delivered through the portal vein that travels directly from the intestine, pancreas, and other abdominal organs. Upon arrival at the liver, the venous blood flows through capillary-like vessels called sinusoids to the hepatocytes, the primary functional cells of the liver. Approximately 60 fluid ounces of blood flows through the liver every minute and is loaded with bacteria, toxic compounds, endotoxins, and antigen-antibody complexes.

- Production and secretion of bile: The liver produces 30 fluid ounces of bile per day. The bile is a carrier for cholesterol and fat-soluble toxins.
- Biotransformation: System of inter-connected enzymes that chemically neutralize toxic compounds.

The Kidneys

There are two main areas of excretion for toxic compounds once they have been biotransformed in the liver: the bile via the feces and the kidneys via the urine. Synthesized by the liver and stored in the gallbladder, bile is a complex fluid that is critical in the detoxification process. The liver uses bile as a way to get rid of waste products. Each day, the liver manufactures approximately one quart of bile. Bile serves as a carrier for many toxic substances that are dumped into the intestines. In the intestines, the bile and its toxic load are absorbed by fiber and excreted.

Optimal kidney health is essential for proper detoxification. The kidneys filter over 150 quarts of blood per day, working to separate the toxins out and eliminate them through the urine. Maintaining a continuous flow of toxins through the kidneys requires adequate amounts of fluid intake to avoid dehydration. Dehydration leads to an accumulation of toxins in the blood, which ultimately affects the function of the kidneys.

The Gastrointestinal Tract

Over a lifetime, the gastrointestinal tract processes more than 25 tons of food, representing the largest load of antigens and xenobiotics confronting the human body. The GI system is the first point of contact for the majority of environmental toxins needing to be further broken down and detoxified from the body. The tips of the microvilli lining the intestinal tract contain a high concentration of detoxification enzymes called CYP3A4. It is this fact that identifies the instrumental role of the GI tract in the process of detoxification.

The gastrointestinal tract receives and processes massive amounts of "external information" and is also a reservoir for several hundreds of species of bacteria and other microbes. These bacteria have the potential to modify hepatic function and overall health. Gut flora can produce compounds that can either inhibit or induce detoxification activities.

When there is an imbalance of bacteria in the gut, substances that pass through the liver and into the intestines for biliary excretion become susceptible to reactivation by bacterial enzymes called beta-glucoronidases. These enzymes revert molecules back to their original form, releasing them back into circulation, a process called enterohepatic circulation. Conversely, microbial enzymes may amplify toxicity in the body. For example, beta-glucuronidase has been observed to be 12.1 times higher in the colon of cancer patients compared to healthy controls.

Other Organs of Detoxification: The Lymphatic System and the Skin

The lymphatic system acts as an elimination route for fluids. It contains large amounts of white blood cells, which monitor the waste in the lymph. This process is so important that without it we would die within 24 hours.

The lymphatic fluid flows into the blood at the insertion of the thoracic duct, into the vena cava as it enters the heart, and is delivered via the blood to the liver for detoxification and elimination.

The sweat glands are a major route of elimination for toxins. At a rate of one pint per hour, the sweat glands produce fluids (perspiration) that serve as a vehicle for the elimination of toxins.

How to Support the Detoxification Systems

A program that is going to support healthy detoxification processes should include the following:

- Removal of all foods that contain toxins and food allergens
- Elimination or reduction of ongoing toxic exposure in the home and/or workplace
- Consumption of a diet rich in whole foods that are filled with vitamins and minerals. Eat only high quality fats and proteins. It takes life to give life, so eat organic or from the source!
- Use of support supplements ONLY when a strong nutritional foundation has been established and ONLY when needed. Supplements can assist in providing specific cofactors required in enzymatic reactions and can protect against the stress hormones. However, if supplements are taken without proper nutrition, they can be turned into toxic metabolites and perpetuate the vicious cycle.

Natural Skin Care

As you begin to clean out your medicine cabinet and rid your life of xenoestrogens and toxins, you'll want to find natural replacements for your skin and beauty regime. Many things that you eat can actually work really well topically, too. In fact, if you can't eat it, I wouldn't put it on your skin!

As mentioned previously, coconut oil is great for your skin. It contains lauric acid, which is anti-microbial, meaning it will kill unhealthy yeast, fungus, and bacteria on your skin.

For a couple of our favorite beauty recipes, try the following:

Natural Face Masks

Removing Blackheads With Gelatin

Step 1: Place 1 tbsp. unflavored gelatin powder in a microwave-safe bowl. Add 1 1/2 tbsp. milk to the powder and mix with a spoon.

Step 2: Set the bowl in the microwave and heat the gelatin mixture for 10 seconds.

Step 3: Dip your fingers into the bowl and coat your face with the gelatin mixture.

Step 4: Leave the gelatin mask on your face for 30 minutes or until it dries completely. The mask will feel stiff when dried.

Step 5: Pull the mask off. As the gelatin comes off the skin, it will take the dirt, dead skin cells, and clogs with it.

www.livestrong.com/article/181015-how-to-remove-blackheads-with-gelatin-milk

How to Make a Mask Using Aspirin

Aspirin is betahydroxy acid (aka salicylic acid or BHA), which is an exfoliant and has anti-inflammatory properties. It causes cells on the epidermis to unstick themselves, thus removing dead cells and allowing regrowth of new skin. It can be used for acne and to improve hyperpigmentation and photo-damaged skin. Most acne products contain BHA.

This mask can be used one to two times per week.

Materials:

- Bottle of aspirin that is uncoated or BC (which is powdered aspirin)
* Avoid all coated aspirin as it takes forever to break down and is coated with colorings, etc.
- Honey: contains enzymes to rejuvenate the skin. Use aloe vera if you are allergic to honey

Process:

Step 1: Take 3 aspirin in your hands OR if using BC powdered aspirin, use one packet in the palm of your hand/or on a plate

Step 2: Add 1 tsp of water on top into your hands; a bit less if not doing this in your hands

Step 3: Let the aspirin dissolve and break down

Step 4: Squirt a few small drops of honey onto the dissolved aspirin

Step 5: Take mixture onto your fingertips and apply to your face (avoid getting it on/in your eyes)

Step 6: Let it sit until it gets hard and dry, approximately fifteen minutes

Step 7: Wash off with water in a circular motion. You might get a tingly effect, which is "the aspirin effect!"

Click here for tutorial.

Conclusion

Slow and Steady Wins the Race
You know the saying, "Nothing good comes easy"? Keep this in mind as you move through this process. Your body is likely in a vulnerable state if you relate to any of the symptoms we've outlined in this book, so going from 0-100 should be avoided. Give yourself space and go slowly. In fact, the slower you go, the more success you will have. Moving too fast can overload the system, which can be completely counterproductive! Reducing the burden on the system quiets the system down so healing can actually happen. **Healing cannot occur in chaos.**

There are many grey areas in this approach, which is why taking notes, getting to know yourself, and reacquainting yourself with your body's language is so important.

How Soon Should I See Results?

How much are you willing to honor and respect your limits and boundaries? How much are you willing to trust the voices in your head or the feeling in your gut? Your body is always sending you messages; are you willing to begin paying attention?

There are many variables when it comes to each individual's healing process: history, age, gender, genetics, belief systems, commitment, job, children, and life experiences. Healing is life-long, but the more attentive you are to your process, the faster you will begin to notice improvements in your energy, a decrease in your symptoms, and, over time, a gradual building of your overall resiliency to stress.

The lesson here is that even though your body is a very complex organism, *you* have control over what happens to it. Greater health and vitality are yours for the taking if you take the time to implement the steps outlined in this book. Take it slowly, listen to your body, and enjoy the process!

Thank You

Thanks for reading *The Female Body Blueprint*. We sincerely hope you enjoyed it and found the information useful for your journey to health.

If you would be so kind, please take just a moment to leave a review of this book on Amazon. As authors, this is a big help to us, and we'd love more than anything for this book to reach as many women as possible. The best way you can help make that happen is to take the time to leave a thoughtful and honest review on Amazon. Please do that now before you get busy doing other things and forget.

Many thanks and best of luck to you in all of your health endeavors,

Josh and Jeanne

The Next Step

We hope you found this information useful and are ready to take the next step for REAL results!

Achieving hormonal balance is no easy feat in this modern day and age. We're up against all kinds of obstacles. Our environment and food supply is filled with chemicals that have an estrogenic effect in the body. Many common pharmaceutical drugs recommended to women commonly are estrogenic as well. To make matters worse, many foods and exercise routines being recommended to women increase the estrogen load even further.

But there's one thing that we have tremendous control over that is the single most important thing for combatting this problem--*making the right nutritional choices*.

For much more extensive and personalized tools to help you optimize your nutrition for stress management, hormonal balance, and metabolic enhancement, we welcome you to our introductory Fight Fatigue with Food Program.

In this course, we will take you step by step through developing a healthy diet specific to your individual needs like no program you've come across before. In addition, we will include some simple (but revolutionary) at-home assessments to help you monitor your success--not just for fighting fatigue, but as the foundation for the precise, cutting-edge medicinal use of nutrition.

Please, come join us here:
(http://www.fightfatiguewithfood.com)

About the Authors

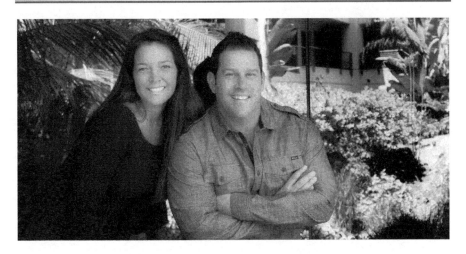

Josh grew up on the East Coast, in Boston, MA, and Jeanne was born and raised on the West Coast in San Diego, California. That's right, California girl meets East Coast boy. They could not have come from two more different backgrounds, but as destiny would have it, they united as EastWest Healing and Performance in 2007.

Their journeys from where they came from to where they are today are just as different as *they* are. Josh grew up an athlete in a very health conscious home, and Jeanne, well, not so much. As the only girl out of five children, affordable food, and enough of it, was the primary goal. None of which supported the severe menstrual cycles, brain fog, extreme mood fluctuations, and low energy she experienced from puberty and into her late 20s.

Josh and Jeanne have spent over 20 years establishing themselves in the fitness and nutrition industry. As authors, mentors, consultants, speakers, and educators to individuals around the world, Josh and Jeanne Rubin pride themselves on their approach to working with the wholeness of each individual and have dedicated their practice to helping people help themselves.

Made in the USA
Middletown, DE
19 August 2015